Anti-Aging

Anti-Aging Secrets
Anti-Aging Medical Breakthroughs
The Best All Natural Methods And Foods To Look Younger And Live Longer

By Ace McCloud
Copyright © 2013

Disclaimer

The information provided in this book is designed to provide helpful information on the subjects discussed. This book is not meant to be used, nor should it be used, to diagnose or treat any medical condition. For diagnosis or treatment of any medical problem, consult your own physician. The publisher and author are not responsible for any specific health or allergy needs that may require medical supervision and are not liable for any damages or negative consequences from any treatment, action, application or preparation, to any person reading or following the information in this book. Any references included are provided for informational purposes only. Readers should be aware that any websites or links listed in this book may change.

Table of Contents

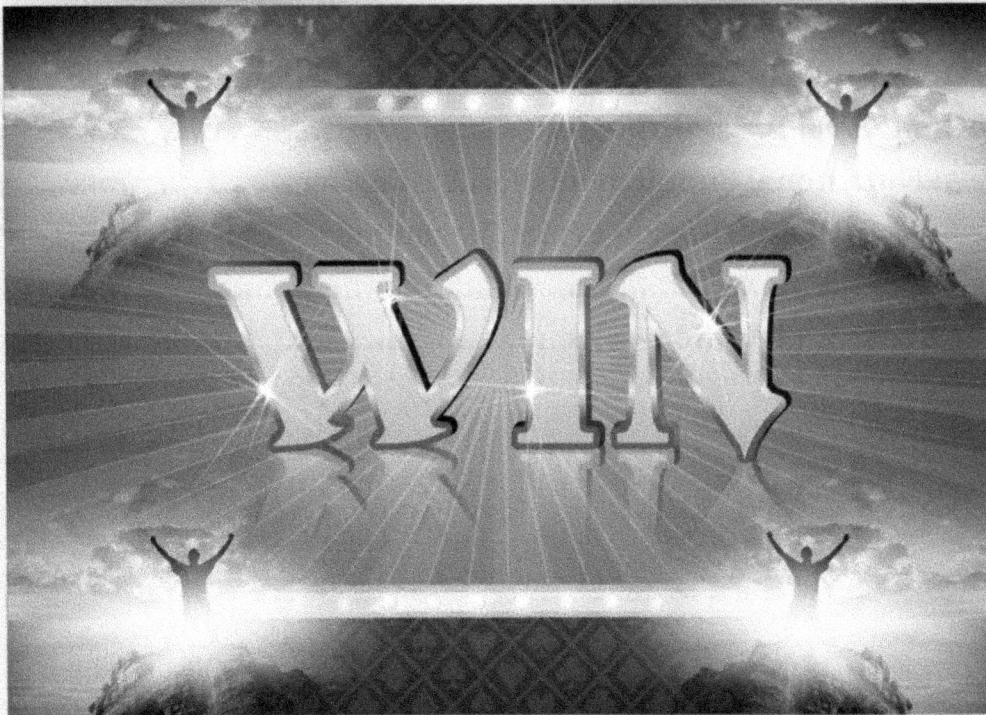

DEDICATED TO THOSE WHO ARE PLAYING THE GAME OF LIFE TO

WIN

KEEP ON PUSHING AND NEVER GIVE UP!

Ace McCloud

Be sure to check out my website for all my Books and Audio books.

www.AcesEbooks.com

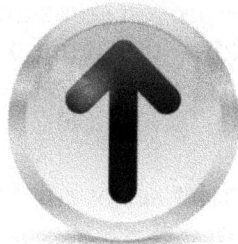

Introduction

I want to thank you and congratulate you for downloading this book. In the following pages you will discover proven steps and strategies on how to fight the signs of aging and how to slow down the aging process. While it is impossible to stop the aging process entirely, it is possible to slow it to a crawl – Hollywood stars have been doing it for years!

This book does not lay down a strict set of rules that you must follow to achieve your desired effects, but rather, makes a series of easy-to-follow suggestions that will make your fight against the effects of aging convenient and enjoyable – without having to spend a small fortune on expensive products and treatments. Slowing down the aging process is not only possible, but it is easy to achieve by following the suggestions and recommendations in this book. Life is so much better when you look healthy and are full of vitality and energy! To discover what you can be doing to live your life to the fullest, keep on reading.

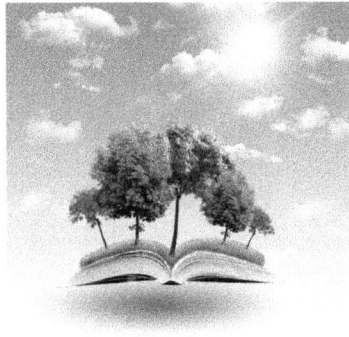

Chapter 1: An Overview of Anti-aging and the Causes of Aging

The Causes of Aging

Let's begin with a simple fact: aging is a natural process that happens to every living thing on this planet. No matter what we try, no matter what we do, from the moment we are born, we get older. It's an inevitable part of life.

The fact that aging is unavoidable is an area for debate among scientific communities, particularly since the isolation and mapping of the human genome. However, despite numerous research attempts to slow down or reverse aging, scientists are unable to prove that aging can be affected by medical means alone.

One fact that scientific communities agree on is that aging is affected by a combination of genetic and environmental factors, the latter of which we have a significant amount of control over. This is good news because it means that our lifestyles have a direct influence on the *rate of aging*.

Anti-aging

Scientific communities are working hard to find medical ways to slow or prevent the aging process. Some scientists are even working on ways of reversing aging. While the future looks promising, scientific research has been unable to provide any definitive answers.

In the meantime, the world marketplace has become full of products whose creators claim can defy the aging process. There are products available that are manufactured by reputable companies who have gone to great lengths in researching and testing their products. However, many manufacturers are unscrupulous and will advertise products without having any research to back up their amazing claims. Before investing in any, oftentimes expensive, anti-aging products, do your own research. Check for reviews on the internet, research the evidence behind a company's claims about their product, and always read the labels on the product you are about to buy.

Chapter 2: Inexpensive or Natural Methods for Looking Young

There are many expensive anti-aging products on the market today. It seems like every other commercial on TV is trying to get us to buy the latest creams, scrubs, pills, and make-up products that will enhance our appearance and make us look more youthful and attractive. In many cases the products are very expensive, and there may be better uses for your money in the anti-aging fight. Here are some affordable and effective things you can do to keep yourself looking younger without investing too much in pricey commercial products:

White sugar

While we typically use white sugar to sweeten our coffee or foods, white sugar makes an excellent exfoliator. The size and hardness of the white sugar helps strip away dead skin cells, which make our skin appear dry and dull.

Consuming refined white sugar assists aging by breaking down collagen, which keeps our skin looking plump and smooth, but, using refined white sugar mixed with your favorite mild cleanser in the bath or shower will improve the smoothness of your skin.

As we age, our body becomes less effective at shedding our dead skin cells, but by mixing white sugar with sufficient quantities of lemon juice to form a rough paste, you can make an affordable skin treatment to help peel away dead skin layers and cells. Lemon juice has the added benefit of containing alpha hydroxy acid – a chemical that is found in many expensive commercial anti-aging products. This acid helps to leave your skin looking smooth and supple.

Keep your eye areas looking great

One of the areas that can make us appear older is the eye area. Wrinkles (often referred to as crow's feet) and dark circles under the eyes are common problems for those of us that wish to retain a more youthful appearance.

Treat your eyes as a separate area from the rest of your face, and don't use anything that is going to irritate the delicate skin around your eyes. For example, lemon juice and sugar is a great all-over body exfoliator, but lemon juice will irritate delicate skin and if it gets in your eyes... ouch!

Keep the skin plump and moist by using a mild moisturizer and exfoliate with cotton balls and warm water. If you wear make-up regularly, keep the layers light and remove nightly. Allowing make-up residues to build up around your eyes is a sure-fire way of speeding up the ageing of your skin.

Here are a few great ways to reduce the appearance of dark circles under the eyes. Take two slices of cucumber or two slices of potato and then place them on your closed eyes. Then take two small bags of ice and hold them over the cucumber or potato slices for several minutes. After doing this for several days you should see some good results.

Another great way to reduce circles under the eyes is to take two caffeinated tea bags and put them in a glass of water. Don't swirl the tea bags around, just put them in the water and then place them in the refrigerator for around 45 minutes. When you are ready, take out the chilled tea bags, lie down, place one tea bag over each eye, and relax that way for twenty minutes.

You can also rub vitamin k cream under the eyes several times per day, as well as Vitamin E. Both of these vitamins will help reduce the appearance of dark circles under the eyes.

Getting good amounts of sleep, drinking lots of water, and also making sure you are taking enough Vitamin C will also help keep your eyes looking great.

It is also very important to make sure your eyebrows are groomed properly. Eliminate any stray hairs that deviate from the natural eye brow line.

If you would like more information on eye and vision care, be sure to check out my book: Eyesight and Vision Cure.

Foundation Make-up

One of the worst offenders for clogging pores and causing build-up on your skin is foundation make-up. Using foundation too often and in too large a quantity often has the opposite effect than the one you desire – flawless skin. While foundation is used to create a blemish-free canvas for you to put your make-up on, it is damaging the skin underneath by not allowing it to breathe and clogging up your pores with harmful residues.

To avoid the aging effects of foundation, don't use it. Instead, use a small amount of concealer to flatten the effect of any blemishes. If you want to add a particular tone to your skin, simply use a tinted moisturizer.

You may simply be unwilling to go without your favorite foundation. If this is the case, only use as much as you need, and use a mild cleanser and cotton balls to remove it nightly, thus preventing harmful make-up residues from building up.

Pay Attention to your Hands

Another area that people notice aging effects the soonest on is their hands. We stretch the skin of our hands so often that collagen breaks down and our skin begins to lose its elasticity. Once the elasticity is gone, wrinkles develop in abundance.

To improve your skin's elasticity, consider exfoliating daily. There are many products out there that claim to help, but many are expensive and don't work very well. An effective and inexpensive recipe is to use is the exfoliating mixture of sugar and lemon we discussed earlier. You can also exchange the lemon juice for olive oil if you want for a more moisturizing effect. Scrub this mixture on your hands, arms. Or anywhere else on your body desired, one to two times per week for best results. If you are a smoker who has developed nicotine stains on your fingers, you will find that the lemon mixture will help reduces the nicotine stains appearance.

There are a variety of ways to moisturize your hands. Aloe Vera gel is always an excellent choice. You can also use almond oil, mineral oil, or a variety of lotions that are on the market.

Another great way to moisturize your hands is to soak them in the following mixture. Fill a bowl with warm water, 5 tablespoons of olive oil, and let your hand soak for around fifteen minutes. When done soaking your hands, lightly rinse them off, pat them dry, and put on your favorite moisturizer. I love Aloe Vera gel, but it can be expensive.

Smoking

One of the leading causes of premature aging is smoking. The effects of smoking on speeding up the aging process seem to be endless. Lung problems, cardiovascular disease, tooth staining – the list of issues goes on and on. If you are serious about trying to reduce the aging process, quitting smoking would be a great start! If you are currently a smoker, then I would highly recommend you read my book: Quit Smoking Now Quickly And Easily.

Coffee and Red Wine

While many love coffee and red wine, both beverages play havoc with the whiteness of your teeth. Yellowing and stained teeth can give you an aged appearance, and is generally considered unattractive. Dark colored sodas and tea can also stain your teeth.

Try brushing your teeth with mashed up strawberries and baking soda every once in a while. The acids in the strawberries break down surface stains on the enamel of your teeth, while the baking powder helps to remove surface plaque and tartar.

Another great trick is to drink beverages like coffee, tea, and wine with a straw. While this may not be ideal, it will protect your teeth from the staining properties of these drinks.

Teeth whitening toothpastes and products are also great for whitening your teeth, just be careful not to overdo it and possibly damage the enamel on your teeth.

Moisturizing

There are hundreds of moisturizers on the market today. Some of them are expensive, some ineffective, but nearly all of them make the claim that they will reduce the effects of aging. Many of the ingredients contained in these moisturizers can be found in products you have around your home.

Buttermilk contains lactic acid, one of the hydroxy acids that decrease the amount of dead skin cells retained by your skin. Soak a washcloth in buttermilk and apply it to your face. Then, rinse gently with warm water so that some of the lactic acid remains on your skin.

Honey is a natural humectant. This means that it draws moisture from the air. If you mix equal parts honey and water, then apply it to your skin, the same effect occurs: the water is drawn to and absorbed by your skin, thereby moisturizing it. Gently rinse after fifteen minutes or so.

A mashed avocado makes a very good moisturizer. The avocado oils are a natural emollient that lubricates the spaces between your skin cells. Furthermore, these oils are readily absorbed by the skin increasing elasticity and giving a smooth appearance. The vitamins contained in avocados also help your skin get rid of dead cells and retain moisture.

While not technically a moisturizing agent, using olive oil on your skin creates a layer of linoleic acid that helps to retain the moisture already contained in your skin. Sesame oil also provides this effect. Also, as mentioned above, 100% Aloe Vera gel, store bought moisturizers, almond oil, and mineral oil can help moisturize and protect the skin as well.

Green Tea and Green Tea Powder

As you may already be aware, green tea is packed with antioxidants. Antioxidants reduce the amount of free radical compounds in your body, which reduces the rate of aging. Try brewing some white tea and then mixing green tea powder into it until a thick paste is formed. Use this as a face mask for twenty minutes, then rinse. You will find that your skin appears plumped, and you will have loaded your skin with a massive dose of antioxidants.

Green tea is also a great drink for anti-aging. The antioxidants and health benefits of green tea have been well researched and documented.

Ginger Tea

Drinking a cup of ginger tea every morning will load your body with gingerol, which is known to reduce the effects of collagen breakdown. As mentioned earlier, collagen breakdown reduces the elasticity of your skin and causes the appearance of wrinkles. Sweeten your ginger tea with honey for extra anti-inflammatory benefits. All natural organic raw honey tends to have the most health benefits.

Chapter 3: Lifestyle Choices That Help Keep You Young

Your lifestyle also plays a huge role in the aging process. Simple changes to your lifestyle can make a huge difference not only in the overall quality of your life, but in the management of your aging process as well.

Sleep

Sleep is vital to a good state of mind and body. Getting a restful night's sleep provides several physical and neurological benefits that are useful in slowing down the rate of aging.

When we sleep, our bodies go into a state of deep relaxation. Our muscles 'slacken', allowing them to rest and heal. This in turn, allows our skin to maintain its elasticity, which is essential in maintaining a more youthful appearance. Long enough periods of sleep reduce 'bags' under your eyes and allow elasticity to return to your facial skin. Similar benefits will be seen all over the body.

A further benefit of getting enough sleep is the positive effect it has on your brain. Research has shown that regularly getting too little sleep builds up a 'sleep debt', which has a detrimental impact on your body's metabolism, increasing the incidence of lowered mood and depression, along with a decrease in overall energy levels.

Sleep can be disturbed by a wide variety of factors. Environmental factors such as outside noise, a room that is too warm or too cold, the type of bed you are sleeping on, or a window that is letting in too much light, can be enough to disrupt healthy sleep patterns. Steps should be taken to address sleep disruption due to environmental factors.

Health factors can also be a concern. Sleep apnea, gastroesophageal reflux disease (GERD), and even snoring can interrupt the necessary relaxation we experience during sleep. If you believe you are suffering sleep deprivation due to health factors such as these, it is important that you speak with your doctor as soon as you can. They will be able to discuss management techniques and treatments that may be available to remedy your lack of sleep or quality of sleep.

The recommended amount of sleep you need to garner maximum benefits varies depending on who you ask, but the general consensus is that anywhere from between seven-and-a-half to ten hours of sleep per night is optimal. It is important to remember that we are all different, and that we all require different amounts of sleep, especially depending on our level of activity or a variety of other factors, so a little bit of experimentation on your part may be required. A rule of thumb is that if you don't wake up feeling refreshed, you didn't get enough sleep. If this happens, a good relaxing nap is a great way to recharge.

I personally switched to a select comfort air bed around ten years ago and it has been one of the best decisions I have ever made. I sleep better, can adjust the firmness, and I no longer wake up with back pain like I used to when I had a regular mattress. They also last an incredibly long time, as long as you can avoid putting a hole in it.

If you are having trouble going to sleep at night, a couple melatonin pills thirty minutes or so before bedtime can help you fall asleep, but try not to do this too often as melatonin can sometimes leave you feeling lethargic in the morning. You can also heat a cup of milk to near boiling, then put in a teaspoon of sugar, and then sprinkle in some nutmeg for a nice soothing drink that will help you fall asleep. You can also try eating a light snack of some of the following foods that will help you fall asleep quicker. Thirty minutes before bed time, try having a snack of one or a few of the following: almonds, flaxseeds, peanuts, walnuts, grapes, oranges, bananas, watermelon, broccoli, cheese, yogurt, low fat ice cream, Kale, corn, spinach, grapefruit, or plums.

Stimulating Body and Mind

Just as it is important to relax our bodies and minds, it is important to stimulate them as well. If you have a particularly hectic lifestyle, it may seem like an impossible feat for you to fit in anything but your daily responsibilities, but, if you want to slow down your rate of aging, you're going to have to find the time to do what is necessary.

Massage and Meditation

Massage is a great body stimulant, and meditation is good for the mind. Try getting your partner to put on some relaxing music, light up a few candles, and give you a back rub or body massage before going to bed. You can use this time to meditate, thus combining the body stimulating effects of the massage with the mind stimulating effects of the meditation. This not only saves you time, it provides a relaxing environment to aid you in falling asleep. If you don't have someone who can give you a massage, then hiring someone is a great option. Although expensive, the therapeutic effects of a professional massage are legendary. If you would like to know more about Massage, Trigger Point, and Acupressure Therapy, then I would highly recommend my book: The Best Of Massage Therapy, Trigger Point Therapy, And Acupressure.

If you would like to see a great guided meditation video, then check out this YouTube video by The Honest Guys: Guided Meditation - Blissful Deep Relaxation. My personal favorite place to get guided meditations and self-improvement downloads is from: Learning Strategies and Hypnosis Downloads.

Mental Stimulation

If you have a little more time on your hands, try stimulating your mind by solving some logic-based puzzles. These will help you 'stay sharp'. If puzzles aren't your thing, try writing some poetry, painting a picture, working on a favorite hobby, or another of your favorite mind intensive activities. The list of things you can do to stimulate your mind is nearly endless, find something that you enjoy doing and try and do it whenever you get the chance to keep your mind sharp. You don't have to be very good at what you are doing – the fact that you are engaging your brain will be stimulation enough to give positive results. When you are bored of a certain activity, move onto something else. Learning something new cannot only be rewarding, but it can help keep your brain sharp as well.

Spirituality

Spirituality is also highly recommended by many anti-aging professionals. This needn't mean going to your local church every Sunday, or converting to a religion you don't believe in. Just having some peaceful time to yourself where you can relax, meditate, and focus on all the good things in life, can help keep you more optimistic and positive about your present and your future. When you are relaxing or meditating, this is a great time to visualize of the completion of some of your various dreams or goals. When used consistently, visualization can have some very beneficial effects on your mind and body. Here is one of my favorite YouTube videos by Jason Stephenson that deals with forgiveness and trying to clear your mind of negative thoughts and emotions: Ho'oponopono Hawaiian Healing Technique Prayer Guided Meditation Visualization.

Yoga

Yoga is great for increasing concentration, along with joint and muscle flexibility. Yoga can be done very inexpensively: some loose clothing, relaxing music, a soft mat, and internet access or a good book are all you need to get going. The library is a great resource for free books and dvd's on yoga. Or you can join a yoga class. This has the added benefit of social interaction, which has been shown to be important in the prevention of degenerative conditions such as Alzheimer's. Here is a great YouTube video by Yoga Shala if you are looking for a beginner's lesson on yoga, Vinyasa Flow Yoga Class for Beginners.

Reducing Stress and Anxiety in Your Life

Stress and Anxiety can be very damaging to your overall health and quality of life. Below are a few great methods and things that you can do to help reduce stress, calm fears, and relieve anxiety. I prefer all natural methods to help solve anxiety problems over the drugs that a typical doctor may try to prescribe for you. You may also want to check out my Laughter Therapy book to bring more joy and happiness into your life. Here are some other great ways to relieve stress and anxiety:

Tai-chi

Tai-Chi is an ancient tradition by the Chinese that was originally used for self-defense. Nowadays, it has already evolved into an exercise that is graceful in nature, and it is used to reduce stress, as well as other health conditions. This is oftentimes described as a type of meditation in motion. Serenity is promoted through the use of gentle, flowing body movements. There are numerous health benefits that practicing tai-chi regularly can bring: It promotes serenity, inner peace, stress reduction, balance, flexibility, fitness, and even helps with heart diseases and eating disorders. Here is a great YouTube video by BodyWisdomTV that shows Tai-chi in action, <u>From BodyWisdom's Tai Chi for Beginners with Chris Pei – Intro, Warm-up & Part 1 Yang 24 form</u>.

Bach Flower Remedies

Bach Flower remedies are another way of treating anxiety naturally. This is a system of 38 Flower Remedies that was discovered more than eighty years ago in England by Dr. Edward Bach. These remedies help to reduce negative emotions by flooding the body with the positive essences gathered from flowers. When used in combination with proper diet and exercise, the remedies can help restore joy and happiness. The essences are wholly intended for self-help at home, and the solutions are diluted in water and should only be taken a few drops at a time. They are not meant to cause a dramatic change or healing, but they can help according to the list of benefits below. Flower essences are safe for pregnant women and children.

Here are some of the flower essences that could be used to alleviate anxiety:

Mimulus: This can be used when a person feels fearful, such as fearful of losing a job, fear of insects, or something of this nature. It is also rumored to help overcome shyness.

Cherry plum: This can be helpful when the mind is stressed or over-strained

Aspen: This is said to be good for when a person is fearful but without a known stimulus. For example: When someone feels like something bad is going to happen, but they have no logical reason to feel this way.

Rock Rose: This is said to help when people experience fright or terror, as well as when they are unable to think or move clearly.

White Chestnut: This is said to be helpful to those who cannot sleep due to a mind cluttered with too many worries and thoughts.

EXERCISE

The most important thing you can do to stay strong, healthy, and fight against the aging process is to exercise regularly. Exercise can be broken down into two main categories: cardiovascular and bodybuilding/weightlifting.

Cardiovascular Exercise

Cardiovascular exercise is absolutely critical in the fight against aging. There are hundreds of ways to boost your heart rate and get your body moving. You can run, walk, swim, play sports, bike, use exercise equipment, join a fitness class, along with a variety of other options. The main thing is to try and get in 20 to 30 minutes of exercise in per day, at least five days a week. If you want to be even healthier, then try for 50 to 60 minutes of cardiovascular exercise per day for at least five days a week. You want to bring your heart rate up and get a sweat going if possible.

The routine that I follow every day consists of the following. After waking up, I drink a big glass of water, jump on a mini trampoline to warm up my muscles, and then I will proceed to casually stretch out all of the main muscle groups in my body. I will then mix up a quick smoothie in my nutribullet blender consisting of only fruits and vegetables. After drinking my healthy drink, I will drink another glass of water along with some vitamin supplements. I then head outside for a nice 30 minute walk. I really like walking because it is extremely healthy, there is almost no chance of injury, and it is a great time to clear your thoughts and just focus on the beautiful things around you. While you are walking, you can also repeat motivational phrases to yourself in your head. I learned this technique from Anthony Robbins in his "Get The Edge" audio CD collection. One of his favorite phrases to repeat is: "Every day in every way I am getting stronger and stronger." Another great phrase that I came up with myself that I like to repeat in my head while walking is: "I am super strong, happy, healthy, wealthy, and pain free." Feel free to make up your own phrase and have fun with it.

The main thing is to make sure you're doing some sort of physical activity almost every day. I could fill the next five pages with all the benefits associated with exercising. The main thing is, if you're truly serious about living a healthy, productive, and long life, you've got to exercise on a continuous basis. No matter your age, it is just something that needs to be done.

Bodybuilding/Weightlifting

Another critical aspect to overall health and well-being is physical strength throughout your entire body. Your quality of life increases dramatically when your body has the strength and power needed to help you live a more enjoyable and healthy life. Not only will you be stronger if you follow a regular weightlifting routine, but you reduce your chances of random injuries and accidents that others who are weaker may fall prey to.

I have been strength training since I was sixteen years old, and it is one of the best habits I have ever gotten into. Muscle burns fat, so if you have a good amount of muscle on your body, it is much easier to stay lean if you are eating a healthy diet. Strength training is also good for your confidence and overall self-esteem. When you are younger, it is much easier to get by without strength training, but as you get older, the effects of a weak body can be downright devastating! Life can be a battle, and if you are weak, it can be merciless. I won't go on to list all the horrible things that can happen to you as you age if you don't strength train, but believe me, it is not a pretty sight! Just look around you the next time you are in public. If you want to live a long time, I would assume you would want to do it with a healthy and strong body. The way I figure it is, the day that I give up on strength training, is basically the day I have given up on life. I highly recommend a strength training routine in everyone's life.

I have had quite a few women talk to me about weightlifting over my life. They are worried that they will get giant muscles and appear masculine. The truth is, it is extremely hard for women to get giant muscles, so if that has been worrying you, then put that worry to rest. A weightlifting routine not only helps men, but women as well, giving them strength and a nice toned appearance that most men find attractive.

Strength Training basics

If you are looking for maximum results, then you want to work out all the major muscle groups each week. If you still want to see results, but don't have the time or discipline necessary for a hard-core routine, then you should make sure your strength training all your major muscle groups in a two-week period. You will also see better results if you do your strength training routine before your cardiovascular training, if you are doing both in the same day.

Before you start to work out, it is always a good idea to take several minutes to stretch out the muscle groups that you will be working. Then, for your first set, this set will always be a warm-up set. That means that you will use light weights and high repetitions to warm up your muscles to help prevent the chance of injury. You always want to do a minimum of three sets per muscle group exercised. If you are doing a hard-core routine, then it is typically five sets. There are many ways to break up your workout routine. The major muscle groups are as follows: legs, chest, back, arms, and shoulders. There are a variety of different programs and exercises to choose from. Find out what works best for you and be consistent!

I personally break up my workout routine into four sections. One day I will do legs, another day arms, another day chest/back, and then finish off with shoulders. I follow this schedule regularly. Typically, I will take one to three days off between workouts, depending on my life schedule and how I'm feeling.

When I was younger, I loved to use lots of weights, push my limits, and see just how big and strong I could get. It was quite exciting, and I got some great results. Arnold Schwarzenegger was one of my role models. However, now that I have entered my 40s, I have adapted a different strategy of using lighter weights and high repetitions so that I have a very small chance of getting injured. I don't have the super muscles that I used to have, but this type of routine has given me a lean, muscular physique that is still very powerful and more than adequate for daily living.

My Strength Training Routine in Detail

Here is the bodybuilding routine that has been extremely effective for me over the last ten years. It is best if you fit all four workouts into a 7 day period, but at minimum all four workouts should be done in a 14 day period, and then just make your strength training routine a habit and never stop doing it. This basic strength training routine has worked great for me, along with a variety of the other exercises mentioned in this book. Also, feel free to mix up the exercises on your own if you are more experienced in order to shock the muscles and stimulate growth.

Leg Day: I will do a short walk around the block to warm up my legs or jump on a mini trampoline to warm up my legs. I will then stretch out my quadriceps, hamstrings, and calf muscles. When properly stretched, I will start off with 25 squats just using my body weight. I go nearly all the way to the ground and I am sure to use good form. I have a Bowflex Revolution, which mimics many of the major exercise machines in a gym. I do light weight leg extensions next to further warm up my legs. After a short rest of a minute or so, then I move on to hamstring curls with light weight and around fifteen or so repetitions. The last exercise will be calf raises. I like to stand on a curb or similar object and just use my calf's to lift up my bodyweight. This completes one full set of all my leg exercises. I then do all these exercises again, only this time; now that I am warmed up, I push myself harder to complete even more repetitions and use more weight. I will then do at least one more complete set of all these exercises, and if I feel like pushing myself, then I will do a complete 4th and 5th set as well. If you are going for power and strength, then after the first warm up set, you want to add more weight and lower the repetitions.

Arm Day: On this day I work out my biceps, triceps, forearms, and grip strength. After stretching out my arms, I will take some lightweight, free weight dumbbells and do arm curls with them until I feel nice burn. I will then take an even lighter dumbbell and do my next exercise, which is for the triceps, called tricep kickbacks. The next exercise is for the forearms, and I will do wrist curls with a dumbbell. I then take a grip strength ball and squeeze it in my hands till I got a nice burn. The last exercise is triceps push downs. At the end of the workout I will typically do a few extra sets of arm curls to really get them strong and looking great. As with all strength training routines, the first set is for warm-up, then you really want to push yourself on the remaining sets.

Chest/Back Day

I start off by stretching my chest and back. I will then take some dumbbells and simulate a bench press motion. When my chest muscles are feeling a bit tired, I end the set with dumbbell flies. I then move to a back exercise, called upright rows. I use a dumbbell with this as well. I will then do another chest exercise called cable crossover on my Bowflex Revolution, and then on to another back exercise called seated rows. I will then do back hyper extensions for my lower back, then some sit-ups, and finish the first complete set with push-ups. Chest back day is typically one of the tougher workouts.

Shoulder Day

I start off by stretching out my shoulders. This routine is done exclusively with lightweight free weight dumbbells. I start the set off with Arnold presses, take a rest, then rear lateral dumbbell raises, then lateral dumbbell raises, and then frontal dumbbell raises. I will then use heavier dumbbells and do shoulder shrugs that work the trapezius muscles. As usual, take a short rest between each exercise.

There a few other things to keep in mind when strength training. You can do your abs and lower back every day, along with your calf's. You can exercise your neck muscles daily as well, and it is good to do various motions with your neck to relieve stress and increase strength. It is also a good idea to eat a protein shake or another healthy food high in protein fifteen to thirty minutes after you have completed your workout.

I hope, in your fight against aging, that you incorporate strength training into it. In my opinion, it is the most important thing you should be doing.

Chapter 4: Medical Breakthroughs

Over the years, scientists and the medical profession have worked on different treatments to slow down the rate of aging. These have included hormone therapies, laser treatments, and dietary supplements. They're not always cheap, nor are they always effective for everyone.

Anti-aging sunscreens contain a compound called Mexoryl XS that blocks harmful UVA and UVB rays from damaging your skin by breaking down the collagen that keeps it looking supple and young. By allowing a build-up of Mexoryl XS on your skin, using these products, eliminates the need for frequent reapplication, giving you protection all the time. La Roche-Posay sells a good product on Amazon called Anthelios SX daily moisturizing cream with Mexoryl XS.

Peptides are found in many commercial products in the drug store or online. These are responsible for boosting collagen production in the skin, thus retaining moisture and plumping the skin, giving a mild Botox-like effect. You can get peptides in an amino form in a supplement, or in a variety of anti-wrinkle and anti-aging creams and lotions. Just make sure that peptides are included in the ingredients of the product.

Wrinkle-filling volumizer injections can reduce wrinkles by introducing a massive boost of collagen underneath a wrinkle, which flattens it out. It is an interesting option because it doesn't paralyze nerves like Botox-type injections. However, treatments costs can be very expensive.

C02 Fractional Laser Therapy is a process in which a laser is used to bore microscopic holes into your skin. This boosts collagen levels, and it is said, by some, to be the most effective anti-wrinkle treatment available on the market today. Its price tag is not for the faint hearted, though. Expect to pay in the region of $5,000 for a treatment like this.

Scientists and doctors agree that the aging process is sped up by decreasing hormone levels in the body, so it's only logical that replacing these hormones would be a good way of slowing down the effects of aging. For men, testosterone has been found to have some pretty incredible effects, and women have found some great benefits from estrogen enhancement. However, hormone replacement therapies have been linked to increased rates of breast cancer and heart attack in some groups of patients. The lifetime cost of hormone replacement therapy varies depending on the length of treatment and fluctuating costs of medications. Talk to your doctor about what options may be available to you.

The FDA hasn't approved Human Growth Hormone therapy for everyone... yet. Currently, it is only approved for people with Human Growth Hormone deficiencies. Costing around $300 per month, HGH therapy is prohibitively expensive to most people, but people that have used it report better mood, muscle tone, and lower levels of body fat. They have also said that they have noticeably firmer skin. Be sure and talk to a doctor before starting a Human Growth Hormone regimen.

Chapter 5: Nutritional Supplements for Anti-aging

When buying a vitamin supplement, it is important to make sure it contains the right balance of vitamins and minerals to boost the effects of your anti-aging regimen. The most important vitamins and minerals to look out for when choosing a supplement are Vitamins <u>A</u>, <u>C</u>, <u>E</u>, <u>K</u>, and <u>Niacin</u>. You also want to use a good multi-vitamin that covers all of the important vitamins and minerals the body needs for optimum performance.

<u>Vitamin A</u> comes in liver, eggs, and oily fish, such as mackerel and tuna. It is an essential vitamin in the fight against aging because it is an antioxidant that reduces the signs of sun damage and reduces the appearance of wrinkles.

<u>Vitamin C</u> boosts collagen levels, which keeps your skin looking youthful and supple, and it also produces sebum, which keeps your hair soft and shiny. Another benefit is that it boosts the effect of all the other antioxidants, so that you get the maximum benefit possible.

<u>Vitamin E</u> is found naturally in leafy vegetables, nuts, and seeds. It is often used as an additive to moisturizers because is help to heal dry, cracked skin. As a vitamin supplement, Vitamin E is an antioxidant that prevents cell damage from free radicals.

<u>Vitamin K</u> helps reduce the appearance of dark circles under the eyes, which are generally caused by leaking capillaries beneath the skin. Vitamins K helps to constrict these capillaries and break up the blood clots that cause dark circles. This vitamin can be found in such foods as spinach and broccoli.

<u>Niacin</u> (or Vitamin B3) is found in many cereals, and it acts as an exfoliant by helping your body shed excess skin cells. Furthermore, as we get older, our skin becomes less able to retain moisture, which leads to dry cracked skin. A regular intake of Niacin assists with our skin's retention of moisture.

Another supplement to try is a fish oil supplement that contains Omega-3. This fatty acid is an excellent anti-inflammatory that help reduce puffy looking skin. It also has the added effect of improving the condition of your brain and acts as an anti-coagulant. There is some evidence to suggest that a regular fish oil supplement reduces the risk of heart attack and stroke. A great product is <u>Kirkland's Omega 3 Natural Fish Oil</u>.

Omega-6 is also an anti-inflammatory. However, most American diets contain far too much of this fatty acid, and people looking to increase the anti-aging effects of their diet typically try to reduce their intake of Omega-6.

In some studies, <u>Grape Seed Extract</u> has been shown to help in the production of collagen and elastin, both of which have a huge positive impact on maintaining healthy skin, hence slowing down the rate of aging.

Resveratrol is commercially produced from the roots of Japanese Knotweed plants that produce stilbenoids when they are under threat from various bacteria. Stilbenoids are an anti-inflammatory, and help reduce blood sugar levels and have an overall positive impact on heart health. While there are no definitive studies on the anti-aging effects of Resveratrol, there is no doubt that it is a beneficial supplement when it comes to cardiovascular health, and something I personally use as well.

There are a variety of supplements that provide the body with the basic building blocks it needs to produce human growth hormone and testosterone. I am not going to recommend any specific products, as they can sometimes have a variety of negative side effects that override their benefits, and they will affect each person differently depending on their diet, lifestyle, and other supplements that they are taking. I can't tell you how many products like this that I have bought in the past, only to have some fairly serious negative side effects, and then find out a few years later that the product was banned by the Food and Drug Administration. If you want to use some of these products, just realize you will need to do a lot of research, and also realize that you may be wasting money on some products that over all do not help you as much as harm you.

A final supplement to mention here is Protandim. This supplement, to date, has not been approved by the FDA to cure or treat any particular illnesses. Its manufacturers claim that Protandim increases the activity of antioxidants in your body, thereby aiding the effect that antioxidants have on harmful free radicals. I have taken this supplement and would recommend it.

Chapter 6: The Best Anti-aging Fruits, Vegetables, and Foods

For the highest quantity of anti-aging effects from food, nothing beats a Mediterranean diet. Increasing your intake of fish, olive oil, whole-grain breads and pastas, red wine, fruits, and vegetables comes highly recommended by doctors, scientists, and nutritionists alike. Not only does a Mediterranean diet increase your overall health and reduce your chances of suffering a heart attack or stroke, it also provides many anti-aging benefits.

Fish

Fish that contain high levels of Omega-3 fatty acids have been shown to have anti-aging benefits. Omega-3 fish oil is an anti-inflammatory agent that reduces puffiness and also reduces the rate at which the DNA in our bodies breaks down, hence prolonging a youthful appearance.

Not all fish contain the same quantities of Omega-3. The fish that contain the highest levels of beneficial oils are mackerel, lake trout, herring, Bluefin tuna, salmon, sturgeon, Albacore tuna, lake whitefish, anchovy, and bluefish. I also like to take an omega 3 supplement to make sure that I am getting enough of this vital nutrient.

Olive Oil

Like Omega-3 fish oils, olive oil contains an anti-inflammatory agent. This is called oleocanthal. If the body and skin is provided with enough of this agent, it has been shown to hold back the aging process. Olive oil is also rich in polyphenols that help protect against and repair damage done to cellular DNA.

Red Wine

Red wine provides several benefits in the fight against aging as it contains polyphenols and tannins. Small quantities of red wine, taken with meals, have also been shown to aid digestion.

Polyphenols have an antioxidant effect on free radicals in the body. By reducing the amount of free radicals, you are actually reducing the negative effects they have on your body, hair, and skin.

The tannins in red wine have been shown to keep you looking more youthful by keeping your skin supple, soft, and smooth.

As with any alcohol, don't drink too much of it as it will begin to have detrimental effects on your health and skin. If you don't drink any alcohol at all, try drinking a cup or two of black grape juice instead. You will still get the polyphenols and tannins, but you won't benefit from the digestive effects.

Whole-grain Breads and Pastas

Eating a diet rich in whole-grains has been shown to keep you heart healthy. This helps retard your rate of aging by keeping your blood vessels in peak condition.

Having a healthy blood flow keeps skin looking healthier and younger by feeding your skin a constant supply of essential anti-aging nutrients.

Another benefit of whole-grain products is that they are high in zinc, which is clinically proven to increase the production of new skin cells. In addition, when eaten regularly, zinc has been shown to reduce outbreaks of acne.

Other Great Anti-Aging Foods

Some more great foods to include in your diet that help in the fight against aging include: Yogurt, Cocoa, All types of Nuts, black beans, Barley, Flax seeds, Oats, Peanut Butter, Ginger, Onions, White Beans, Sweet Potatoes, Dark Chocolate, Mushrooms, and Green Tea.

Fruits and Vegetables

The many benefits of a regular diet filled with fruits and vegetable has been highly recommended by governments, scientists, nutritionists, and the media for decades. They are also a huge part of the Mediterranean diet. Colorful fruits and vegetables are typically the ones that provide the highest levels of anti-aging benefits.

Tomatoes are a huge source of lycopene, which act as a natural skin protectant against ultra-violet rays. Over time, a diet rich in lycopene can reduce the appearance of wrinkles and skin cell damage. When tomatoes are cooked, the lycopene levels are increased, which makes tomato-based pasta sauces a perfect choice in the fight against aging skin.

Garlic is a great source of antioxidants that help reduce damage caused to cells by free radicals in the body. Black garlic contains double the amount of antioxidants as regular garlic, so try using this in your cooking for maximum anti-aging effect. If you're worried about the smell of garlic on your clothes and your breath, try removing the little green shoot inside each clove. This will reduce the odor significantly.

Bell peppers contain large doses of Vitamin C, which boosts collagen levels in your skin. Higher collagen levels fight the appearance of crow's feet and wrinkles, and helps keep the skin looking smooth. As a rule of thumb, the closer to red that a bell pepper is, the more Vitamin C it contains and the sweeter it tastes.

Spinach is another rich source of Vitamin C. Another benefit of a high intake of Vitamin C in your diet is the fact that it helps your body produce a compound known as sebum, which helps hair look healthy and shiny.

Romaine lettuce is packed with more nutrients than the typical iceberg lettuce we all know and love. Just as crispy, Romaine lettuce contains high levels of Vitamin A, which is essential for new skin growth and the expulsion of dead skin cells. This process helps fight wrinkles and helps keep skin looking refreshed.

Zucchini contains silica in its peel, which helps boost collagen levels in your skin.

Some more great fruits and vegetables to include in your diet in the fight against aging include: Blue berries, Broccoli, Grapes, Apples, Cherries, Guavas, Kale, Pomegranates, Goji Berries, Carrots, Kiwis, and Pineapples.

While this is by no means a complete list of beneficial fruits and vegetables, it will serve as a nice go to list for the next time you're pushing a shopping cart around the grocery store wondering what to buy.

A Super Anti-aging Recipe

Here is a super-easy, super-tasty, super anti-aging recipe. It is a typical recipe that would be served in the Mediterranean, and it incorporates many of the ingredients you have just read about. If you don't drink alcohol, don't worry, we're going to boil that off and just leave the beautiful, rich flavors.

Here's what you'll need:

1 Carrot, diced small

1 Onion, finely chopped

3-4 Cloves of Black Garlic, peeled and crushed

1 tbsp. Olive Oil

1 Small Glass of Red Wine

1 Small Glass of Water

1-2 tbsp. Tomato Paste

1 Red Bell Pepper, deseeded and chopped

4 Tomatoes, deseeded and cut into chunks

1 Large Handful of Cherry Tomatoes

5-6 Fresh Basil Leaves, finely chopped

2 Medium Zucchinis, washed and thickly sliced

2 Large Handfuls of Baby Spinach Leaves, washed

1 Vegetable Bouillon Cube

As much whole-wheat pasta as you need

Here's what you need to do:

1. Gently sauté your carrot, onion, and garlic in the olive oil until soft.
2. Add the basil and continue to sauté for one minute.
3. Remove these ingredients to a separate bowl.
4. Crank up the heat until the pan is very hot, then pour in the red wine. It will sizzle, and it will be loud. Let the wine simmer until the smell of alcohol disappears.

5. Add in the contents of the bowl, the tomato paste, the water, the bell pepper, the four tomatoes (save the cherry tomatoes until later), the zucchini, and crumble in the bouillon cube.

6. Let this mixture simmer until it begins to thicken.

7. Finally, cook your pasta to your desired taste, and add your spinach leaves and cherry tomatoes to your sauce. Remove from the heat as soon as the cherry tomatoes begin to split, and the spinach leaves are wilted.

8. Serve, and enjoy!

Juicing and Smoothies

One of the best things I did to improve my overall health was to regularly include juicing and smoothies into my diet! I have been using a Juicer the last five years and absolutely love it. A great juicer is the: Breville Juice Fountain. I also just got a NutriBullet Blender recently and am very pleased with that as well. Incorporating both juicing and smoothies into your diet is a great way to fight against the aging process, and get your body tons of easily digestible vitamins, minerals, and nutrients! There are hundreds of recipes out there, with a million ways of combining every sort of vegetable, fruit, and healthy ingredient for a nearly unlimited amount of ways to make healthy smoothies and juices. I would recommend just taking your favorite anti-aging foods from the list above and then juicing them or making a nice smoothie. It really does not need to be an exact science, and honestly, just about every juice drink and smoothie I make with fruits and vegetables tastes pretty good to me.

This is what I will do on a typical day when I am eating for maximum anti-aging and peak performance. In the morning I make a smoothie of only fruits and vegetables. The reason for this is that fruits and vegetables will digest much quicker if you do not have any other proteins with them. My favorite ingredients to use are: Spinach, pineapple, green peppers, apples, oranges, bananas, grapes, strawberries, celery, kale, and carrots. Two to three hours later, after I have had my morning walk, I will eat a small meal of almonds, sunflower seeds, and peanuts. The majority of the nuts I eat is almonds, however, as they tend to be the healthiest and give the most energy.

Three or four hours later I will have a regular dinner, and then at night, an hour or two after dinner, I will make a nice juice drink with a huge variety of fruits and vegetables from the list above. I just cut up all the fruits and vegetables, run them through the juicer, and get about a quart of juice. I then spend the next thirty minutes or so drinking it, as it is best consumed quickly after juicing for maximum benefit. I like to juice after dinner, because if you juice on an empty stomach, it can cause significant pain in your stomach sometimes. You can also juice less amounts of fruits and vegetables if you want to be more economical. At night, around an hour or so before bed time, I will have another light snack or smoothie. Smoothies are great for getting all the foods in your system digested and incredible for keeping you regular. The same goes for juicing as well. I have found that smoothies are much less expensive and time consuming, while juicing takes a significantly more amount of time and money, but really gives you that added boost of energy that you may be looking for.

Conclusion

While there are many products in the marketplace, it must be accepted that aging happens. It's inevitable. Yet we must also accept that there are many things we can do about the rate of aging. Diet, exercise, lifestyle, and environmental factors all play a part in how quickly we begin to show the signs of aging and how successful we are at slowing it down. While we can't reverse the aging process, making small changes to how we live out our lives can have a massive impact on how youthful we look and feel.

I hope this book was able to help you to take a look at some easy ways to make changes to your lifestyle and diet that will have a beneficial impact on your rate of aging. I also hope that you use the knowledge gained in this book to improve the quality of your life.

The next step is to implement some of the things that you have learned into your life. Try some of them for a couple of weeks, and keep a diary in which you can write down any improvements that you notice. Keep doing what works for you. With a serious effort, you should be able to add years onto your life, with increased energy, strength, and improved appearance!

Finally, if you discovered at least one thing that has helped you or that you think would be beneficial to someone else, be sure to take a few seconds to easily post a quick positive review. As an author, your positive feedback is desperately needed. Your highly valuable five star reviews are like a river of golden joy flowing through a sunny forest of mighty trees and beautiful flowers! *To do your good deed in making the world a better place by helping others with your valuable insight, just leave a nice review.*

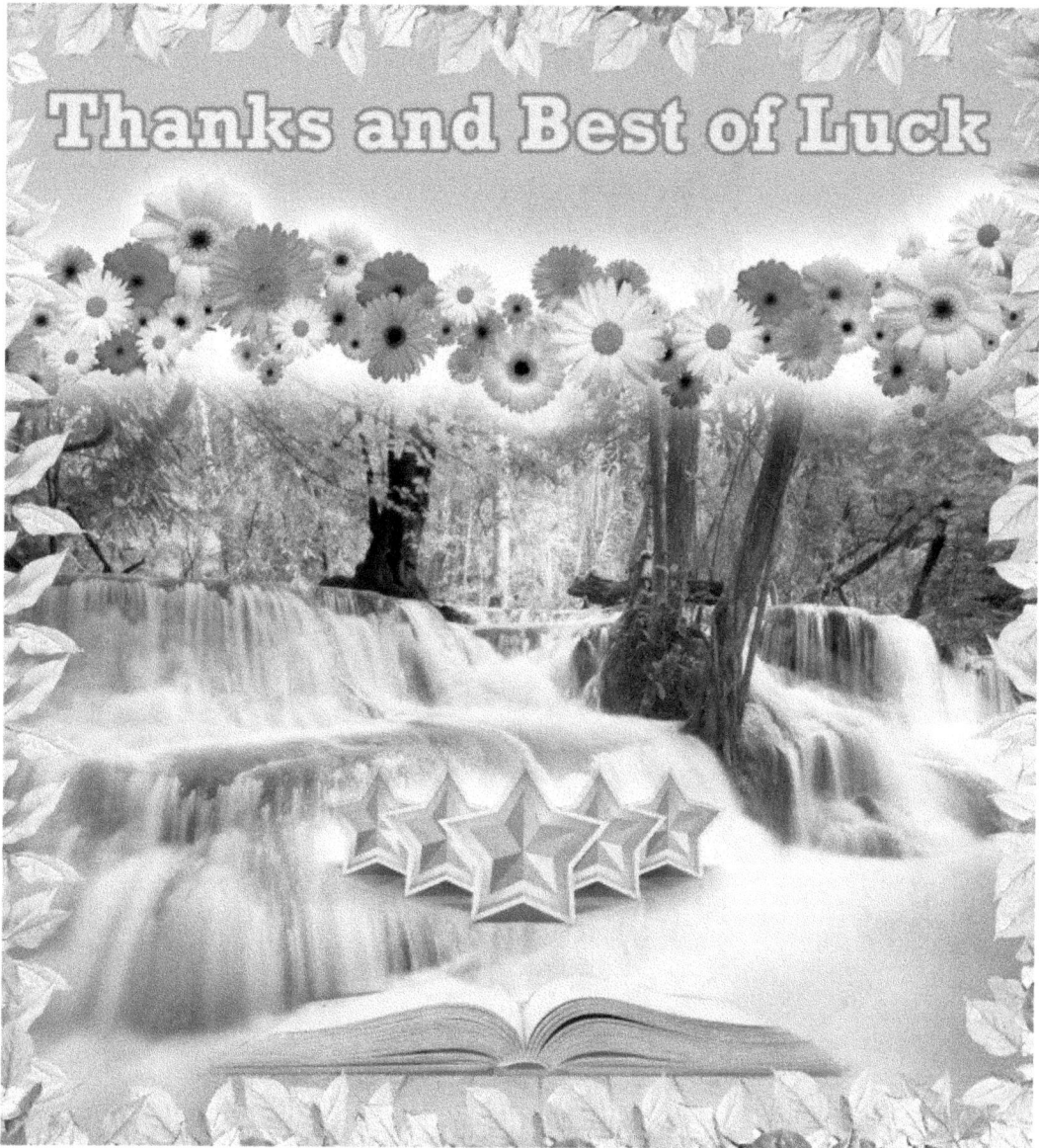

My Other Books and Audio Books
www.AcesEbooks.com

Health Books

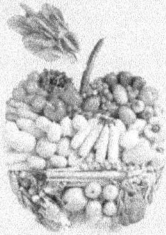

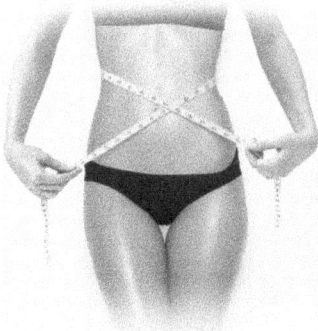

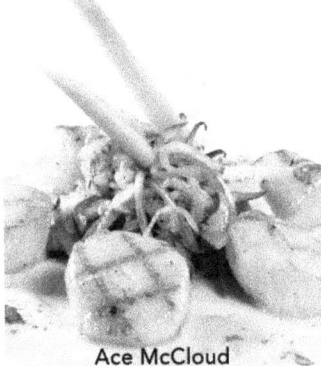

Peak Performance Books

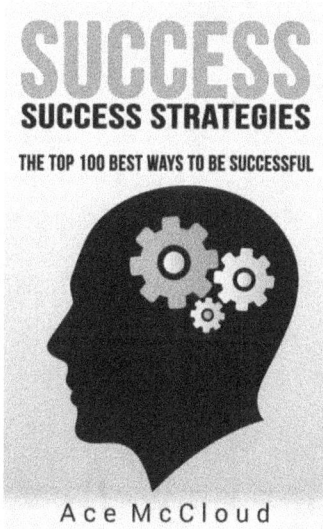

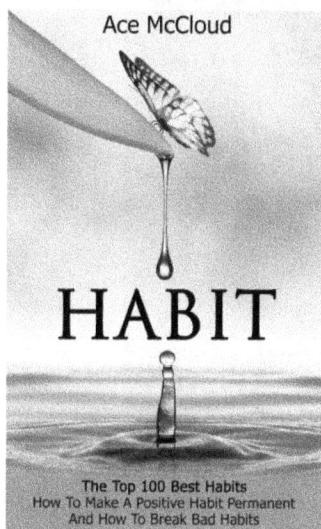

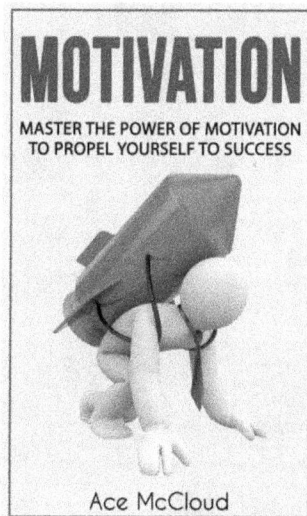

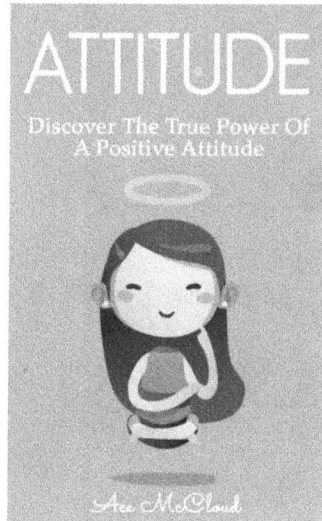

SUCCESS
SUCCESS STRATEGIES
THE TOP 100 BEST WAYS TO BE SUCCESSFUL

Ace McCloud

Ace McCloud

HABIT

The Top 100 Best Habits
How To Make A Positive Habit Permanent
And How To Break Bad Habits

MOTIVATION
MASTER THE POWER OF MOTIVATION
TO PROPEL YOURSELF TO SUCCESS

Ace McCloud

ATTITUDE
Discover The True Power Of
A Positive Attitude

Ace McCloud

SELF DISCIPLINE

Unleash The Power Of Self Discipline, Influence And Willpower In Your Life To Achieve Anything

Ace McCloud

Competitive Strategies
WINNING STRATEGIES

The Top 100 Best Strategies For Peak Performance During Competitions

Ace McCloud

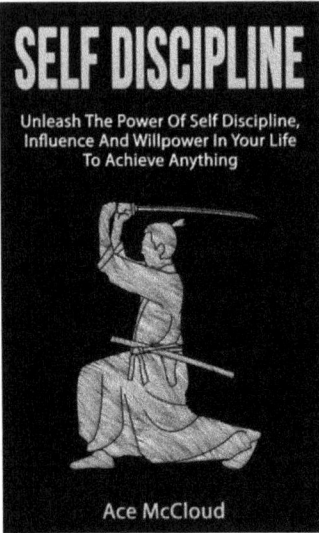

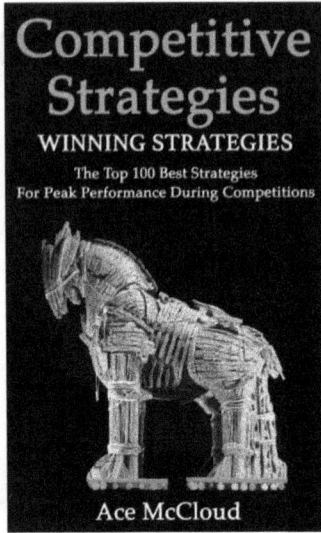

Be sure to check out my audio books as well!

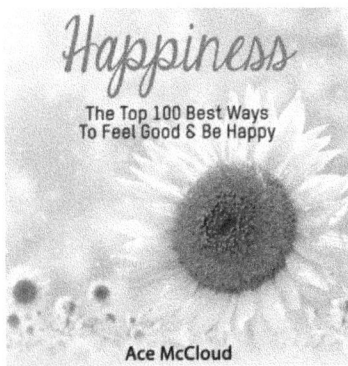

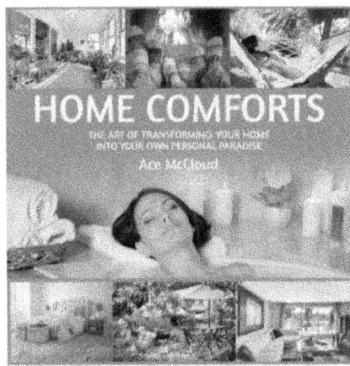

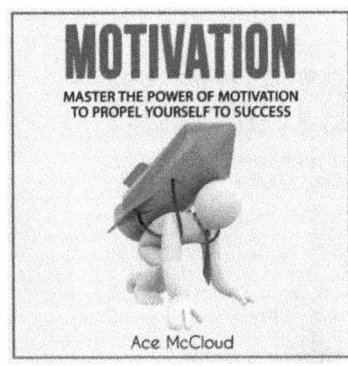

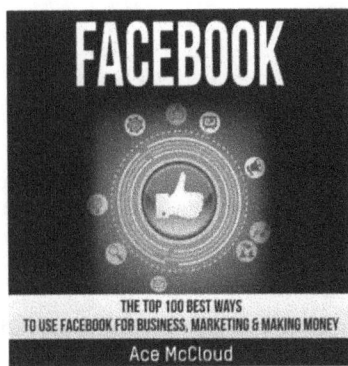

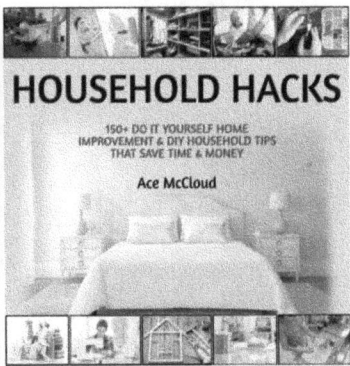

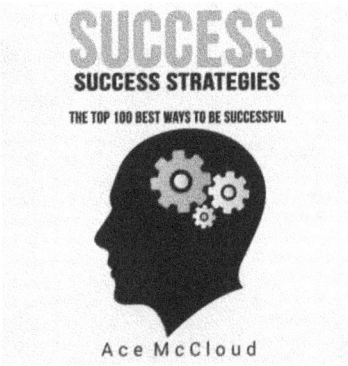

Happiness

The Top 100 Best Ways To Feel Good & Be Happy

Ace McCloud

HOME COMFORTS

THE ART OF TRANSFORMING YOUR HOME INTO YOUR OWN PERSONAL PARADISE

Ace McCloud

MOTIVATION

MASTER THE POWER OF MOTIVATION TO PROPEL YOURSELF TO SUCCESS

Ace McCloud

FACEBOOK

THE TOP 100 BEST WAYS
TO USE FACEBOOK FOR BUSINESS, MARKETING & MAKING MONEY

Ace McCloud

HOUSEHOLD HACKS

150+ DO IT YOURSELF HOME IMPROVEMENT & DIY HOUSEHOLD TIPS THAT SAVE TIME & MONEY

Ace McCloud

SUCCESS
SUCCESS STRATEGIES

THE TOP 100 BEST WAYS TO BE SUCCESSFUL

Ace McCloud

Check out my website at: www.AcesEbooks.com for a complete list of all of my books and high quality audio books. I enjoy bringing you the best knowledge in the world and wish you the best in using this information to make your journey through life better and more enjoyable! **Best of luck to you!**

www.ingramcontent.com/pod-product-compliance
Lightning Source LLC
Chambersburg PA
CBHW080632030426
42336CB00018B/3173